M000042108

WEIGHT LOSS SURGERY:

THE REAL SKINNY

BY

NICK NICHOLSON, M.D.

AND

B.A. BLACKWOOD

PUBLISHER'S NOTE

This is a compilation of observations and conclusions made and drawn during many years of treating and performing surgery upon bariatric patients by W.D. Nicholson, IV, M.D. It does not, and does not purport to, give medical advice to the reader, although hopefully it will be useful to those contemplating the use of bariatric surgery to lose weight.

Published through the generous support of

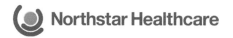 Northstar Healthcare

Copyright © 2014 Nick Nicholson M.D. & B.A. Blackwood
All rights reserved.

ISBN: 0615887392
ISBN 13: 9780615887395

Library of Congress Control Number: 2013950824
Obesity Resources Publishing
Dallas, TX

Acknowledgements

The publication of this book would not have been possible without the generosity and support of Northstar Healthcare Surgery Center Dallas to whom I express my most sincere thanks.

Nick Nicholson, M.D.

Table of Contents

CHAPTER ONE

Weight Loss Surgery – Punching The Reset Button

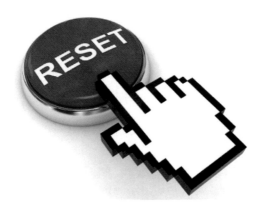

Did you ever wish you could go back in time ten, twenty or thirty years and just start over on your weight battle? Before you had to buy a seatbelt extender or take medication for high blood pressure or stay home because you couldn't climb the bleachers to go to your son's football game? Back when you only had twenty or thirty pounds to lose, not 120 or 130 pounds?

If you could just punch a reset button and start over, you know you'd have a fighting chance to stay at a healthy weight, a chance you don't seem to get no matter how many diets you try or how hard you work at it.

That's what weight loss surgery does. It takes the steering wheel, hits the gas, and accelerates you at warp speed to a weight that had always before seemed hopelessly out of reach. It's the ultimate do-over, just like Bill Murray in the movie *Groundhog Day*. But unlike the movie, you won't get multiple chances to get it right.

As the pounds come off, emotions will break loose that you never even knew were there, not only in yourself, but in your friends, family and co-workers. If you're not prepared for them, the emotional tide can overwhelm you, sabotaging your weight loss and undoing the physical changes your surgeon made to your body.

Most patients never dreamed that the simple loss of weight could create such turmoil.

> *"The hardest thing for me has been dealing with all the emotional issues. You can bet that whatever has been eating you is going to surface. I didn't realize it then, but I was stuffing things. Numbing emotions. I feel everything more intensely now. I'm glad I did it [had surgery] even though it was like ripping off a band aid."*

> *"It never occurred to me that other things in my life would change. I just wanted to get healthy. But it affected everything – my marriage, my kids, even my job."*

"My husband started out being very supportive. He even paid for my surgery because my insurance wouldn't cover it. But then he started making nasty comments about my weight loss. He got mad whenever I left the house wearing makeup. If someone would say something nice to me about how I looked, he'd say something derogatory."

"Some of my friends don't want to go out with me anymore. Before, I'd been the funny fat girl who could get the guys to come over so my friends could flirt with them. After I lost the weight, the guys wanted to keep talking to me, and my friends didn't like that."

"People who'd never spoken to me at work suddenly started being nice to me. I wasn't mad at them before the surgery, but now I'm really angry at them. It's all I can do just to say hello."

Why is being prepared for this emotional backlash important? Because overeating has little to do with physical need and everything to do with emotional need.

The truth is that obesity cannot be surgically "cured". Weight loss surgery isn't some sort of permanent dietary prison lockdown. Even the most drastic bariatric procedure can be undone by an unwillingness to adapt to a healthier way of life. Its purpose is to give you a fresh start and a period of time to adjust to a new lifestyle regimen under optimum conditions. It'll be up to you to carry those new habits forward after the seeming magic of the operation has worn off.

In other words, bariatric surgery gives you a winning edge, like being given a ten mile head start in a 26.2 mile marathon race. Whether you wring every benefit out of that head start and win the race or decide to squander that precious advantage by heading to the showers after mile eleven is totally up to you.

Your relationships with friends and family will change because of your weight loss. Emotions will boil to the surface that may surprise you, and not necessarily in a good way.

To win the weight loss marathon, you're going to have to learn to deal appropriately with the intense emotions that will bombard you after the surgery. If you don't, you'll fall victim to "head hunger" - eating for reasons wholly unrelated to hunger or need - and wind up right back where you started, staring at your bathroom scale like it's the messenger of doom.

Most patients aren't aware they have an emotional Achilles' heel until it smacks them in the face right in the middle of their weight loss. So if you don't know what emotions your surgery and diminishing size will provoke, how can you be ready to deal with them successfully?

That's what this book is about. It helps you recognize your own emotional landmines so that you can defuse them before they have a chance to wipe out your weight loss efforts.

Scared? Don't be. The emotional "reveal" from the surgery can be as healing and joyful as the weight loss itself.

If you handle the emotional issues that arise in a healthy way, your life can be better than your most optimistic hope when you stepped into your surgeon's office.

CHAPTER TWO

How Did I End Up In This Mess and Why Can't I Get Out of It?

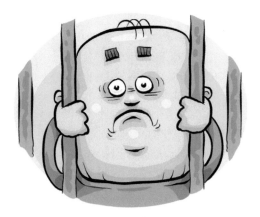

Maybe you've been heavy your whole life, or you never lost the pregnancy weight, or the pounds your high school football coach was ecstatic about when you were his star lineman have morphed into less muscle and more fat. One day you look around and realize that you're bigger than most of the people around you. You know you're not perfect, but it doesn't seem that you eat that much differently than everyone else.

How in the world did you end up as this super-sized version of yourself?

Most people don't become obese by binge eating or a thyroid problem. Weight gain can be unnervingly insidious and usually comes from eating anywhere from 10 to 100 calories more than you need per day.

Yes, you read those numbers right – just 10 to 100 calories a day.

If you eat the equivalent of one Life Saver, only 10 calories, over your body's caloric needs every day, you'll have gained a pound by the end of a year. Increase those extra calories to 100 a day, and you'll be ten pounds heavier than you were just a year before.

If you keep it up for ten years, you'll step on the scale finding that you've gained a staggering one hundred pounds. That's why you can wake up at 40 thinking you haven't really been eating that much to find that you've crossed the line into obesity.

Most people have no idea how overweight they are until something bad or embarrassing happens. It's as though your mind's eye protects you from seeing yourself as you really are up until the moment when your doctor tells you that you have diabetes or you see a photo of yourself at the company picnic.

"I was at a party with my husband and realized I was the biggest woman there, including a lady who'd had a baby just five days before."

"My friends and I had to walk a few blocks to get to a restaurant. By the time we got there I was

sweaty and out of breath, and they were all fine. I was so embarrassed."

"I went to a meeting with potential clients and couldn't fit in the chair at the conference table. That was it for me."

"I went with my friends to an all-you-can-eat sushi bar and we sat together at one table. We're all pretty heavy. I looked around and noticed other people in the restaurant staring at us like we were a bunch of pigs. I had to get out of there. I didn't want to be part of that group anymore."

Whatever inciting event led to your decision, the day comes when you resolve that you're going to lose the weight. Period. You go on a diet and drop three sizes, but then go back up four. You try a different diet. Same result. You combine exercise with yet another diet. No luck.

You rarely lose as much as you'd like, and the pounds you manage to carve off seem to come back in less time than it took to lose them.

By the time you consider bariatric surgery, you've probably tried at least ten diets. You may have tried extreme liquid diets or "sensible" diets like Weight Watchers or Jenny Craig. But no matter how hard you tried, the end result was the same.

It's little wonder that by the time you walk into a bariatric surgeon's office, you feel like the extra weight you're carrying around is lit up in red lights blinking "FAILURE" visible from a mile away.

> *"I've been on a diet since I was eight years old. Believe me, I'd tried them all. I felt like the biggest loser in the world. Why did it seem so easy for everyone else?"*

> *"I was thin in college and really active. But after the kids were born, I could never lose the weight no matter what I did. I just kept getting bigger and bigger. I hated the way I looked, but I couldn't seem to lose the weight."*

> *"I'd lost forty pounds on Weight Watchers but then couldn't lose anymore. Losing it and then not being able to lose anymore and gaining it back was worse than never having lost the weight at all. I just felt hopeless."*

> *"I went on a liquid diet for three months and looked better than I ever had in my life. But the second I started eating real food I gained weight. It all came back almost as fast as I'd taken it off."*

Why can't you lose down to a healthy weight and stay there? Why are you such a failure as a dieter?

Actually, you're probably a champion dieter. The problem is that you're fighting a losing battle with your own physiology.

Hunger fits right up there on the scale of physiological needs with air and thirst. In other words, your need to satisfy hunger is just as strong as your need to breathe or to drink water after you've been outside in the heat. It's impossible to repress that need for extended periods of time, but when you have a lot of weight to lose, that's exactly what you're asking your body to do.

Even Superman couldn't win that battle.

Here's how it works. Ghrelin is a hormone that tells you when you're hungry. When its levels are high, you're hungry. Once you eat, your ghrelin level goes back down, and then rises again as the food digests. This is what the ghrelin levels look like for a non-dieting person at a healthy weight who eats three meals a day:

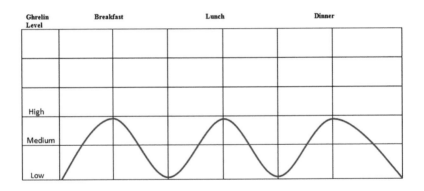

Now, let's say you need to lose a hundred pounds and you go on a sensible 1200 calorie a day diet designed to result in a one pound per week weight loss. The red line below represents your ghrelin levels:

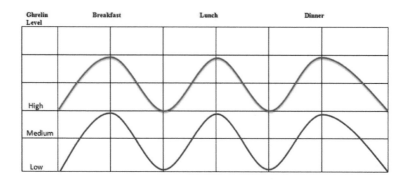

See the problem? At the fullest level, your ghrelin levels never drop below the hunger level that would drive an average weight person to the refrigerator. In other words, your fullest sensation on your sensible diet is equal to the hungriest sensation of a non-dieting person at a healthy weight. No wonder so many people on a diet complain that they're always hungry. They are.

To lose one hundred pounds, you'd have to maintain the 1200 calorie a day diet perfectly for 23 months – 734 days – a feat requiring more than just discipline and desire. It requires hand to hand combat with physiology that's screaming "feed me, feed me, feed me" at you every hour of the day.

It would be the same as telling someone who's just spent two hours mowing the lawn under a sweltering sun that they can't have a drink of water and repeat that every day for 734 days in a row.

The gastric bypass and gastric sleeve surgeries avoid the part of the stomach called the gastric fundus which produces ghrelin.[1] In other words, they take the hunger hormone off your back so that your diet can work.

---

1 This does not apply to the lap band procedure, which is solely a portion control operation.

The green and orange lines below represent what the ghrelin levels look like for anywhere from six to eighteen months after the gastric bypass and gastric sleeve surgeries:

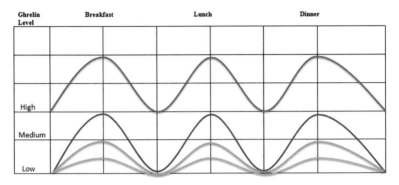

For a time, the ghrelin levels following surgery won't even reach the hunger level of a non-dieting person. This won't last forever, and other hormones will eventually come into play to make up for the lower ghrelin levels. However, the surgeries can trick your physiology for long enough to allow you to lose a significant amount of weight, giving you time to get in the behavior modification groove of less food, more exercise, and the development of habits designed to last you the rest of your life.

Lowering ghrelin levels won't address your head hunger but it's a useful tool. During the six to nine month period of maximum ghrelin suppression you'll learn what it feels like to "need" food versus "want" food. You'll be at the controls of your own biofeedback laboratory, getting the knack of reading the signals your body sends you when it's low on glucose and needs fuel without the noise of a faulty ghrelin message clouding the communication.

So, back to the 10 to 100 calorie a day example. You got to an unhealthy weight a little at a time. You could theoretically lose the weight 10 to 100 calories at a time, but that would only take off 1 to 10 pounds a year which isn't going to resolve your weight-related health problems in a timely manner, nor is it impressive enough to give you the motivation to stay the course.

With the 1200 calorie a day diet, you can shed pounds faster, but fighting your physiology every day for the length of time it would take to lose the weight is unlikely. Your inability to lose the excess weight and keep it off is predictable and inevitable.

What does this all mean?

You're striving for a permanent weight loss that's near impossible. It's no wonder that morbidly obese people have a 98% failure rate for lasting weight loss through non-surgical diet methods.

You're not a failure – you just haven't been given the right tool. Bariatric surgery isn't easy, but most of you have already proven that you have the discipline and desire to lose weight. Your issue is losing enough weight and keeping it off.

That means you're exactly the type of person that weight loss surgery can help.

CHAPTER THREE

Talking To Your Surgeon: No Time to Practice Lying

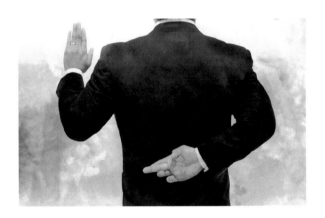

The instant you choose a specific weight loss surgery, you've begun setting the odds for success or failure, just like a handicapper at the betting counter of the Kentucky Derby. You do not want to be the 30 to 1 odds dark horse in the race.

The three main bariatric procedures – gastric bypass, gastric vertical sleeve and the lap band – all have different effects.

All three can be cheated. All three are simply tools to help you lose weight. All three will work, but only if the person wielding the tool – you – handle it properly, which means you need to select the surgery that gives you the best possibility for success taking into account your own personal characteristics.

Choosing the right procedure should be done with the same care and analysis that da Vinci used in selecting the brushes to paint the Mona Lisa or that Arnold Palmer used to select the golf clubs he won his Masters Tournaments with. The selection demands deliberate, educated, mindful consideration.

Some patients sabotage their odds of successful weight loss by lying at the very beginning, both to themselves and to their surgeons. They don't set out to purposefully lie; rather, the lie comes out as wishful thinking, or what they believe they ought to say to be a "good" patient, or what they envision they'll be like after undergoing surgery.

Don't do it. Nothing less than rigorous honesty will work.

Watch out for these four common lies patients tell themselves:

1. The Variation on the Chicken and the Egg Lie

"If I'm going to spend money out of my own pocket to get this thing done, then there's no way I'm going to mess it up."

"Are you kidding me? I'm scared to death of being cut on and being put under. If I'm willing to do that, then I know I'm willing to do whatever it takes after the surgery."

"I hate pain. I'd be an idiot to risk gaining the weight back after going through the discomfort of the surgery."

"My mom is a nervous wreck about this surgery. There's no way I won't make this work because I'd never put her through this again."

All of these statements have one common fallacy: they assume that if someone is willing to spend money, be cut on, suffer pain, or worry relatives, surely they'll be ready to do everything else necessary to ensure their success.

In other words, if there's an egg, there must be a chicken.

In this scenario, it really does matter which came first, because if you haven't bought into the lifestyle changes required for the surgery to be a success, these outward badges of willingness don't mean a thing.

Every bariatric surgeon has heard a hundred variations of the chicken and egg lie. While most patients make these kind of comments sincerely, the reality is these facts alone won't keep them from going back to unhealthy eating or lifestyles.

Don't make that mistake.

You're going to need every weapon in your arsenal to stay the course, and choosing the right surgery is one of the biggest weapons you have to deploy.

2. The "But I'm Going to do Everything Else Right" Lie

"My favorite foods have always been sweets and I love ice cream. I chose the lap band and didn't

end up losing much weight, and I gained it all back and more. Looking back, I think I chose the lap band because it still let me have sweets."

You might be tempted to choose the type of surgery based upon leaving yourself the option of eating your favorite guilty pleasure food. After all, you're going to be eating smaller portions, selecting healthy food 90% of the time and exercising – all daunting life changes – so why take away your favorite food in the world?

Because it's your trigger food.

Because it leads you to eating more than you should.

Because it will sabotage your weight loss efforts.

Because it will make you feel defeated.

Because it will be the undoing of your weight loss surgery.

It's analogous to a recovering alcoholic recently discharged from the Betty Ford Clinic who swears he'll only drink on special occasions. The clinic staff knows he'll be back for a repeat visit, probably within a matter of weeks.

Choosing a bariatric procedure that doesn't inhibit eating your trigger foods at the outset will doom your weight loss effort. If you find yourself leaning toward a specific procedure because it will allow you to have foods that have always been a problem for you, then your brain may be sending you a signal that you're not quite ready for the surgery.

Listen to it.

3. The Escape Pod Lie

"I decided on the lap band because it doesn't have to be permanent. I don't think it's good

for my body to do something to it that's not reversible. It just seems like that would be unhealthy."

Some patients gravitate toward a particular procedure solely because it's reversible, telling themselves, "Hey, I can always undo this if I don't like it. It's good to have options, right?"

Wrong.

If you're already contemplating reversal of the procedure, that should send up red flags in your mind about whether you're ready for the life change you're about to undertake. In other words, if you go into the surgery already looking for a way out, the chances are you'll sabotage the surgery by your conduct.

If you're ready for the surgery, you'll be willing to lock the door to the escape pod and burn the key for scrap metal.

4. The "But I'm Being Financially Responsible" Lie

"Money doesn't grow on trees. They're all weight loss surgeries designed to help you lose weight. It only makes sense to pick the cheapest one."

We're told to look for the best financial deal from the time we're old enough to understand money. That's usually good advice, but not when choosing the best type of bariatric surgery for yourself. Although it sounds risky to take finances out of the equation, it's far riskier not to. If you pick the wrong surgery, there's a good chance you'll not only have wasted your money on the initial procedure, but you'll have to spend more money on a revised procedure, something both financially and emotionally debilitating.

After you've subjected yourself to a searching inquiry, it's time to pass that information on to your surgeon. He or she will ask you questions like:

- What do you define as success in your weight loss - is it fitting into a size 6 dress or losing just enough to get rid of your Type II diabetes?
- What kind of foods do you eat – sugar, carbs, salty foods, carbonated beverages?
- What unhealthy foods do you have the most trouble resisting?
- How much weight do you have to lose and how quickly do you want to lose it?
- Does your schedule allow twice a month visits to your doctor (required by the lap band), and, even if it does, are you willing to keep that kind of commitment?
- What kind of support system do you have?

There's no right or wrong answer to any of the questions, and there's nothing to be afraid of. Most bariatric surgeons are in the profession because they have a profound compassion for people struggling with obesity, and they're not going to be shocked by anything you have to say. Being honest about your eating habits, your feelings toward food and what's going on in your life will help your surgeon recommend the right surgery for you.

Here's a summary of the three basic procedures, their characteristics, and success rates using national statistics:

	Gastric Bypass	Gastric Sleeve	Lap Band
Amount of excess weight loss[2] at one year	70-77%	55%	36 - 40%
Amount of excess weight loss at 2 years	77%	70%	40-50%
Amount of weight loss maintained after 5 years	65-70% of excess weight lost	65%	60%
Percent of patients who see cure or improvement in diabetes	96%	80-93%	77%
Percent of patients who see cure or improvement in high blood pressure	90%	75%	70%
Ghrelin suppression	Yes	Yes	No
Difficulty in eating processed sugar (dumping syndrome)	Yes	No	No
Portion control	Yes	Yes	Yes
Malabsorption (not absorbing as many calories in small intestine)	Yes	No	No

Although bariatric surgery can sound drastic, the procedure itself can be as safe as gall bladder surgery, a Caesarean section, or having your appendix removed. On the other hand, the risk of not doing anything about your weight can be deadly.

---

2 Excess weight is the amount of weight over your ideal body weight. For example, if you weigh 250 pounds and your ideal weight is 150 pounds, you'd have 100 pounds of excess weight.

Obesity is the second leading cause of preventable death in the United States, and is responsible for 500,000 deaths per year. It increases your risk dramatically for Type II diabetes, stroke, renal failure, high blood pressure, certain types of cancer, congestive heart failure, acid reflux, degenerative joint disease, sleep apnea, certain anxiety disorders, depression, and a host of other ailments.

Whatever reservations you may have about bariatric surgery, you can check the risk analysis off of your list.

But all the good reasons in the world can't give you the desire necessary to have the surgery and do the work you need to maintain the weight loss. That can only come from you, and your willingness to be honest with yourself and your surgeon can give you a quick litmus test of whether you're ready for the procedure or not.

If you can do that, you've just made yourself an odds-on winner right out of the gate.

CHAPTER FOUR

So What's Really Eating You - Get Ready to Find Out

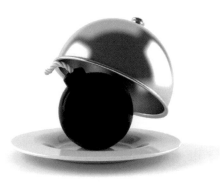

You've made it through the first few weeks, you're feeling good, the scale is suddenly your friend and people are falling all over themselves to compliment you on your new look. But you're overwhelmed by feelings of anger or sadness or fear. What's going on?

"The day I was supposed to go see my doc for a checkup, I had a flat tire. I was ranting and raving like a lunatic. I even slammed my hand on my desk so hard I bruised my pinky pretty badly. I thought OMG if anyone would have just seen that tirade I would have been locked away."

"I feel raw. I can be on top of the world one second and sobbing the next."

"I woke up from my gastric bypass a depressed person with acute anxiety attacks every morning that lasted for hours. The weight was just falling off me, and I could care less. Talk about a disconnect."

"I'm having strange mood swings. I am usually not easily made angry, but I've started going to half days at the office in order not to start crap. I feel like the surgery has brought out the ugly in me."

"I'm fighting a lot with my son. I feel like a snare trap, just waiting for the first person to trip it."

For many patients, weight has been the preoccupying worry of their lives. It's been responsible for their diabetes, their high blood pressure and their trips to the orthopedic doctor for worn-out joints. It's limited their clothes shopping to specialty stores, subjected them to not-quite-under-their-breath scathing comments from airplane seatmates, and stalled them on their climb up the corporate ladder. It's been responsible for their divorce or their failure to get married.

So it's no surprise that the thought of winning the weight loss battle takes on mythic proportions, right up there with finding the Holy Grail. The movie reel playing in your head of life after successful bariatric surgery shows someone whose whole world gets better, an adult version of a "happily ever after" ending.

The reality is rarely as golden as the movie footage. Whatever emotions were masked by your weight, they'll leap to the forefront at warp speed. The job you hate, the parents who never seem satisfied with you, the bad marriage, the rebellious teenager sulking in your home, the buried feelings of unworthiness, the childhood trauma – they're all still there.

And if you didn't know what your emotional hot spot was before the surgery, it will announce itself with a bang shortly afterwards. It's as though your extra weight acted as camouflage, and without it, all your other problems loom as raw and irritating as a mouthful of fiery canker sores.

> *"I wasn't expecting all the emotional stuff. It's scary as hell. That's been the hardest thing for me. Whatever you haven't dealt with, it'll come up."*

> *"I didn't realize it before, but I was just stuffing all my emotions down as I was stuffing food down."*

> *"I stayed in graduate school forever, working on my thesis. I'd been kind of heavy before, but*

in graduate school I really went over the top. I think it was because I was afraid I couldn't make it on my own in the real world. Looking back, I realize I'd gotten that negative message from my mother. I don't know if she meant to do it or not, but I always had the sense that she didn't think I could really take care of myself."

"My whole family is heavy. That's who we are. I didn't think I could ever be anything different. I think I was afraid to be something different."

"I always had a feeling that I didn't measure up, probably because I had an absentee dad who I rarely saw."

"My dad told my mom I was too big when I was nine years old. I was 5'6" tall and weighed 130 pounds so, looking back, I was actually proportionate – just tall for my age. But I've been on a diet of some sort ever since then, and I'm sure that had something to do with where I ended up."

"I spent my whole life trying to please other people, like that was the only way anyone would like me. I guess I didn't really think I was worth taking care of."

"I hear my grandmother's voice in my head telling me 'eat that, it will make you feel better.' I've been doing that my whole life."

"My mother told me I was fat when I was four years old. I've got a lot of shame about food. Whether I'm eating healthy or not, I always feel a lot of shame when I eat."

Some patients have even darker issues to deal with such as sexual abuse or extreme trauma. But the results are the same. People use food as a coping mechanism to soothe, numb, or hide.

Confronting issues you've avoided your whole life will be scary, but the alternative is worse. You can't successfully lose or maintain your weight loss if you continue to use food as a coping mechanism for your life. Surgery will keep you from turning to food for a while, but sooner or later, you'll be back in full control of your eating, capable of sabotaging whatever type of surgery you've had.

You don't want to go there.

The intensified emotions you may feel in the first few months after your surgery are giving you feedback, showing you what issues are eating you up inside. For example, many formerly easy-going patients find themselves rocked by a staggering amount of anger that erupts in seemingly innocuous situations. They may not know what's making them angry, but their subconscious is giving them an unequivocal, insistent message that there's something unresolved they need to address.

Support groups, one-on-one therapy, behavior modification groups, quality reading on the topic – all of these can help guide you through interpreting and dealing with the wave of unexpected feelings that may engulf you after surgery, and your surgeon should have these resources available for you.

Use whatever works for you, but do not ignore the vital input your emotions are giving you.

"My dad was hardly ever around. He hasn't even called me since the surgery. I realized that I'm still seeking his approval and it's never going to come. I had to accept that he's not a good dad and I had to forgive him for that."

"I'm trying not to be so hard on myself."

"I took care of everyone else, but never took care of myself. If I don't do it, who will? Now I'm more focused on what makes me happy."

"I try to be more open. I was kind of stand-offish, hard to get to know. It was really because I was afraid. I still get scared but I really push myself now to be more social. It gets easier every time, and now I realize I'm worth getting to know."

"I was really angry. For me, it was my living situation. I had to make a change."

"I married someone who was just like my dad. I never could please either one of them. I'm now living on my own and working with a therapist on having relationships that are healthy for me."

"I never lost the weight after I got pregnant and just kept gaining. I thought being a good mom meant spending all my time on my children and none on myself. I'm doing what I need to do now to take care of myself, even if that means spending less time with my kids. I still feel guilty about it, but I'm working on that."

"I grazed my way through the day at work. I'd snack all morning and start thinking about what I was going to have for lunch by 9:30 a.m. When I went back to work after the surgery, I got really depressed. I finally figured out that I hated my job and I had to make a change."

"My life was just out of balance. It was all about work. Since I traveled, work let me avoid everything else. I'm trying to balance my life now into thirds – a third for me, a third for my job and a third for my family."

Hard though it may be, facing your problems head on will ultimately give you a better shot at your fairy tale ending. Every obese person has a long and varied emotional road map created by parents, social norms, invisible childhood cues, trauma and the cards dealt by life along the way. The reasons you abuse food may be different from anyone else and may be frustratingly opaque.

That doesn't matter.

The solution boils down to this: figure out what's causing you stress and change it, or, if you can't, find a different, healthier coping mechanism.

Your surgeon can operate on your stomach. It's up to you to operate on your head.

CHAPTER FIVE

What Have I Done to Myself? The Immediate Aftermath

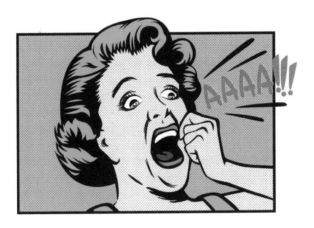

You can't wait to start your new life, the one where you don't have diabetes, you're off your blood pressure medication, you can shop for clothes at a regular store and you can walk as far as you want. You've researched your surgery and know what to expect in the first few days, weeks and months. You did everything you were supposed to do to get ready. So why do you wake up from surgery feeling like you just made the biggest mistake of your life?

> *"If a friend weren't here with me, I'm not sure what I would do. I'm not really in much pain, but I just feel like an emotional wreck. I can't believe I chose to do this."*

> *"The first four weeks were really hard. You're sore, your whole middle hurts, it's difficult to get around. I started asking myself, 'What have I done? Will I ever be the same?'"*

No matter how much you prepare, you'll probably have several days or even weeks of second-guessing yourself about your decision to have the surgery, and this doubt can lead to full blown panic since, at least for the moment, the surgery can't be taken back. It's done. No matter how much you thought you wanted it, the initial reality can be frightening.

What causes patients the most anxiety? It depends on the person, but the reason usually has to do with being stripped of a long time coping mechanism in one fell swoop.

Two-thirds of all bariatric surgery candidates use food as a crutch. It's been their steady companion through break-ups, job disappointments, family stress, anger, loneliness, and even just plain old boredom. Food also acts as the centerpiece of celebratory events – birthdays, promotions, holidays, tail-gating, the start of baseball season, a friend's engagement.

In other words, most bariatric patients use food as a way to deal with emotions, either by numbing them, diverting them, or celebrating them. The majority of their eating has nothing to do with hunger, and an astounding number of patients don't realize just how much food has infiltrated every aspect of their life until they wake up after surgery.

If you're one of those people, you may break out into a cold sweat when the reality slaps you in the face that you can't use your go-to method of dealing with stress at a moment that, let's face it, is really stressful. It's no wonder many people push the panic button.

For patients who've had the gastric sleeve or gastric bypass, the finality of what they've done will hit home with a thud.

> *"For the first few weeks I couldn't even think about the logistics of what had been done to my plumbing or I'd get sick."*

> *"How could I have done this to myself? I can barely take in a sip of water."*

> *"I've turned myself into a freak."*

For all patients, there's the fear that they're going to mess up the operation. Most have been told that if they don't follow the post-surgery instructions to the letter for the first few weeks after the surgery, they could cause severe complications and even die.

> *"I hurt so much right after the surgery. What was I thinking? And then I was freaking out*

about staying on a liquid diet for three weeks. I'd already been on one for two weeks before the surgery, and right afterward I couldn't imagine that I could make it."

"I worried the whole time I was just doing the liquids that once I started getting to eat real food I wouldn't know when to stop. I was afraid I wouldn't be able to feel if I was full, and I'd unknowingly hurt myself."

For others, the realization that they literally can't eat, or even drink like they used to, causes extreme anxiety.

"The one healthy thing I did was drink water. I loved to gulp water. After the surgery I could barely take in a small sip."

"Ten days after the surgery (gastric bypass) I wanted to eat. I wasn't hungry but all I could think about was eating. I tried to take in a little too much liquid and it came right back up. I started bawling."

"The first three weeks were torture. Food was everywhere. My wife was eating in front of me and I couldn't have anything but liquids. I counted forty commercials for food in a one hour T.V. program. I'd never been more conscious of food in my life."

"I wasn't hungry, but my mind was hungry. All I could think about was my favorite steakhouse and how I'd never be able to go there again. At that moment, none of it seemed worth it."

Further, mastering your new system's mechanics in the first few weeks and months can be daunting.

"I threw up a lot. I never knew how I'd react to food. Something I'd eat one day would make me throw up the next."

"Certain foods make my stomach sore, like cabbage or broccoli, and others just make me sick, like avocados. I ate an avocado and felt like I was going to die."

"My friend had the surgery and I tried to eat what she said worked for her. Some of the stuff she eats made me violently ill."

"I had to go to the bathroom constantly."

Dealing with the finality, the restrictions, the fact that you don't feel well, and creating a new user manual for your stomach without the use of your favorite coping mechanism can send some people over an emotional cliff.

"I had many moments of 'what was I thinking?'. I went into a deep depression."

"The first three months were hell."

"I wasn't really myself. I was extremely irritable, and I'm not usually like that. I think I was way too hard on my wife. It's a wonder she didn't leave me."

There's no easy fix for dealing with the anxiety. It's part of the process, and you can take some comfort in knowing that everyone goes through it. Your doctor and support groups, both online and in person, can provide you with help in developing new coping mechanisms and reassurance that this phase will pass.

And it will.

Most patients settle into the new reality between one and three months, and some even sooner.

"The first four weeks were the hardest. After that, I started feeling a bit better, and when I stepped on the scales and saw how much I'd lost, I felt a LOT better."

"It took about three months before I decided I hadn't made a mistake. I had some complications, but I had a friend who'd done the surgery who just kept telling me to ride it out, that it would be worth it. And I did. I'd do it all over again in a heartbeat."

"I didn't feel well for the first month. But then I was able to start moving around more and my

energy level came back up. I started switching to solid foods and figuring out what worked. It just became part of a routine. I began feeling more in control of myself and my body than I had in a long time."

Just hang tight. It'll get better.

CHAPTER SIX

You Enlisted But Your Spouse Was Drafted: The Impact of Weight Loss Surgery On Your Marriage

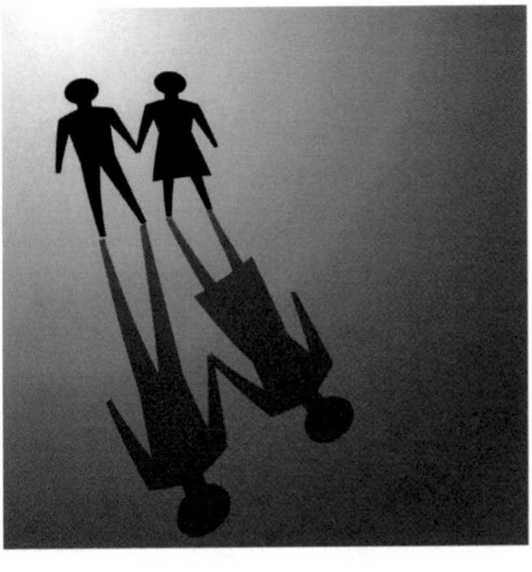

You're changing your eating habits, you're exercising like a fiend, and you're figuring out new ways to deal with the stress in your life. You've changed your job or your work schedule, you're more outgoing, and you're taking greater pains with your appearance. Total strangers are giving you a second look and you're gaining confidence by the day. Your spouse is just as elated as you are, right?

That depends.

Not only is your body changing, but your habits, activities and attitude about yourself are changing too. You can't undergo that kind of evolution without impacting your marriage, which is why the divorce rate for bariatric surgery patients is higher than the national average.

Whether your spouse is happy with the new you, or whether the new you is happy with your old spouse, depends on how healthy your marriage was before the surgery. Bad marriages tend to get worse, good marriages tend to get better, and even perfect marriages will show cracks under the strain of adjustment.

It's as though your marriage will undergo a stress test, and the results will be as clear to both of you as an ECG readout is to a cardiologist. The problems can be minor, such as a temporary adjustment issue, or major, such as an evaluation of whether you can stay healthy and remain in the marriage.

Even the best unions will have to go through an acclimation period. You're changing years-long habits as well as your own and others' perceptions of you, all of which will affect your spouse as well.

In other words, you can't wave goodbye and send your mate postcards of your weight loss journey. He or she will be forced to go with you, and many leave for the trip having packed none of the necessary accoutrements.

Your new lifestyle will require practical changes that your spouse may initially resist. If you and your husband spent weekends researching and trying out new restaurants, you'll have to think of something else to do. If you ate out every night, you'll now be eating in far more often. If your wife's idea of a holiday was touring the Napa Valley wineries, she may not be thrilled with your new vacation ideas. If you're now spending an hour in the gym after work every day when you used to be home helping with the kids, that may cause resentment.

> *"Our life used to revolve around going out to eat. My wife didn't like the change."*

> *"Now I work out every night and do long runs or bike rides on the weekends. My wife was initially supportive, but I think now she's not so sure it's a good thing. I know it makes her take on a bigger load at home, but I have to exercise."*

> *"My wife and I were both foodies. Now I'm not a foodie and she still is. It's a problem."*

Besides the change in your old routines, your spouse will also have to adjust to the unaccustomed attention you may now receive from the opposite sex. Not only will you look more attractive, you'll feel more attractive, which translates into a powerful "I'm sexy and I know it" aura as visible as the marquee lights on a Broadway sign.

For many partners, this raises the specter that you may no longer be attracted to them. They're used to living with a partner who was overweight and unhappy about it, so the threat of a femme fatale or lothario stealing you away had never made it onto their things-I-have-to-worry-about checklist.

The more compliments you receive, the more your spouse may wonder if you'll be content to stay with them. Their insecurity can often be expressed as criticism. It's a crude but understandable technique. After all, if you don't feel good about yourself, you're less likely to leave them for someone else.

"My husband and I pulled into our driveway, and our neighbor was in his yard. He hadn't seen me in a while, and he came over and hugged me and told me how good I looked. My husband said, 'Yeah, but she's going bald.'"

"After I lost the weight, men started noticing me, but my husband didn't notice me at all. He never said a word about my weight loss and just looked at me like I was imagining things if I ever talked about it."

"My husband paid for my surgery because my insurance wouldn't cover it. But now that I've lost all the weight, he criticizes me all the time."

"My wife wanted me to have the surgery, but now says I'm too self-absorbed and that I'll never look like I did when we first met because of my ugly 'skin flab'."

"I got so much attention from other men. My husband wasn't happy about it. He told me he liked me better when I was heavier because he doesn't like my saggy skin."

*"My husband tells me I'm vain. He says I look in
the mirror too much."*

Exacerbating things further, it's only natural to take pleasure in decorating your new self. You may change your hairstyle, dress up more, and display an interest in clothes shopping that your spouse has never seen. Your mate could interpret your new preoccupation with your looks as your way of advertising for his or her replacement.

> *"Watching me go from morbidly obese to 125 pounds was incredibly difficult for my husband. He had only ever known me as puffy. And it wasn't helped by the fact that I had a sense of pride in the slimmer me so I didn't slouch around in sweats, I wore make-up, and I did my hair and nails. He started going everywhere with me. I'd even be at work and find him popping in, saying he was 'just passing by'."*

> *"Skirts got shorter, shirts got lower, and I got a boob job. I wasn't interested in other men, but I can see how he'd think I was. Looking back, I'm aware of how I changed."*

Then there are the spouses who are fighting their own weight problem, and your success can make them feel uncomfortable. You're living proof that weight loss is achievable, and your very presence can act as a constant reproach, highlighting their own failure.

"My wife was supposed to get the surgery too. She kept making excuses and wouldn't keep any of her appointments. She tells me I've changed and she's not sure she wants to be married to me anymore."

"I don't know how my 25 year marriage will turn out. I was the one in shape when we got married. My wife was always overweight. Ever since my surgery my wife is acting distant from me. I am getting back in shape like I was before we were married and she doesn't seem to want to take the journey with me. I get a strong feeling she resents me now."

"I think my wife is intimidated by my will power. She's yo-yo dieted throughout our entire marriage, and has never been happy with her weight. She's been very quiet."

"This weekend we went out and I had planned what I was going to eat, and that's what I had. My husband ordered his usual things and then sat there and talked about how I was making him look like a pig, eating everything in sight."

Your spouse may even work to derail your efforts, trying to get life back to the old comfort zone.

"My wife and I were supposed to do the surgery together. She ended up not following through,

and it was almost as though she was trying to sabotage me. She'd eat everything I was not supposed to eat, like chips, right in front of me and was always telling me it wouldn't hurt to have a little. My wife wasn't committed. She said she was, but she wasn't."

"My wife will cook things she knows aren't good for me, and then roll her eyes at me when I choose to eat something else, as if to say 'surely you can eat that'."

"My husband started out as supportive, but now claims I'm selfish. He says I never cook anymore, which isn't true, and says I'll never stick to my exercise program."

"Our new issue is him having me pick what he's going to eat. It's not healthy food either. He has me ride along to fast food places where he gets burgers and tater tots. He likes to get pizza and have me hold it, and he buys a lot of potato chips and soda. It's hard to watch him eat that stuff in front of me. I can't figure out if he's being mean or just clueless."

Don't panic if your spouse takes a while to get on board with your redesigned self. It's an immutable fact right up there with Newton's law of gravity that no one likes change. Your spouse's discomfort with the accommodations they must make, your new attitude and behaviors, and the attention others pay to you may cause friction. But, in a healthy marriage, all of these problems can be worked through with understanding, communication, effort and the passage of time. Just be patient, and realize that their world is altering almost as much as yours.

"My wife was really resentful about all the time I spent working out in the evenings. I moved my workouts to early mornings before she and my son get up. That helped a lot."

"We went to counseling together and it helped. My wife finally began to appreciate that my weight loss was helping her too. I can now help around the house, which I couldn't do before. I can now get life insurance, which benefits her."

"My husband was very supportive and still is. We had to change a lot of things but it was worth it. We had a good marriage before. It's better now because I feel better about myself."

"My wife wasn't on board at the beginning and was really hard to deal with about the whole thing. She's never had a weight problem and was afraid of the surgery. Now I've got the energy to go and do things with her and she's very happy that I did it."

"We had a great relationship before and we continue to have a great relationship. It is just

different now. I never did outdoor things before, but last weekend we bought a Harley for us to ride. We've figured out other things to do."

If the problems in your marriage that emerged after your bariatric surgery just won't go away despite your best efforts, they may be symptoms of more serious issues.

For many, the weight loss and confidence it engenders causes a power shift in the marriage, revealing fault lines that simply can't be fixed. If you've always gone along with whatever your spouse wanted to do, playing a submissive role in the marriage, neither you nor your spouse may be able to carve out a working relationship based on the new dynamic.

If the cornerstone of your marriage was an unhealthy co-dependence on food or enabling behavior from your spouse, it's unlikely he or she can make the leap with you to a healthier relationship.

If you've tolerated an abusive or loveless marriage, you may decide you have to leave in order to take better care of yourself.

"I got divorced. I'd actually wanted a divorce five years earlier. I never should have married the man in the first place. After I lost the weight, I went through with it. I just decided getting out of that relationship was part of taking care of myself."

"I think the thing the surgery does most is to pull the fat blanket off so you really have to look at your relationship. When I finally looked at him and thought to myself 'I would rather die alone

than live with you,' I knew I was done. I'd been married for 27 years."

"I've told my husband I love him, I want him, but I don't need him. I'm not willing to go back to living the way I was."

"My wife was for me getting the surgery, but now she says I've changed and she wants a divorce. I have changed. I'm more confident, more outgoing, I want to do more things. She'd rather sit on the couch, watch T.V. and snack all night, which is what I used to do. She doesn't want anything to change. I've been out of the house now for two months and I'm already happier. I feel like I have a second chance."

"Other men were telling me how good I looked and my husband never complimented me. In fact, he told me he hated the way my skin looked. The attention from men was overwhelming to me. I'd never had attention like that before. I ended up having an affair with someone who told me I was gorgeous and didn't even notice my skin. My husband filed for divorce. I didn't want it initially, but as time passed I realized it was better for me that he did. He wasn't going to stop being hateful until I regained all my weight, and I'm not going back there."

"In the beginning my husband was very supportive of my surgery, but then he started acting funny. He seemed really distant and very irritable. Next thing I knew, he told me he'd put in for a job transfer and that he was going to move without me. I thought with my weight loss we'd have so much fun doing things that I hadn't been able to do before. I guess he didn't want to do those things. I guess he liked me the way I was before."

"I used to be so quiet and cooperative. Now I'm very outspoken. I actually have an opinion. My husband didn't like it. We ended up getting divorced."

"My husband and I have been having problems. We tried talking about it and he said, 'wow, you're becoming conceited'. I hope I'm not, but I guess it's possible. For over a decade the pendulum has been over on the self-loathing, no-self-esteem side. It would make some sense that the pendulum would swing a little over on the opposite side before settling in the proper place in the middle. I expect that could be part of this process, and that's fine with me. I'm not sure that my husband is going to be able to handle it, though."

"My husband and I divorced about six months after my surgery and he is now dating a woman

who is almost as heavy as I used to be. Even though he said at the time it would be nice for me to lose the weight, we just kept moving farther and farther apart. Maybe it was more secure for him when I was so big."

For most bariatric patients who've been doing time in an unhealthy marriage, they're surprised to find that escaping it can feel as welcome as a governor's pardon for someone on death row. But what if you wanted to stay married and your spouse headed for the exit door?

It hurts. No question it will be hard. But if he or she couldn't handle the new you, whether because of your weight loss, your hard won self-confidence, your insistence on spending time on yourself, or their own irreparable insecurity, then they probably did you a favor.

The alternative would almost always be to go back to the way you were – unhealthy, inactive and cutting your life span short by years if not decades. If that's what you have to do to save the marriage, it's not worth saving.

And your spouse's decampment can open up new, better possibilities.

"My husband left me after I lost about 90 pounds. I think he thought he would leave me before I left him. I was a wreck. Now I'm down to a size 6 and he wants me back. Too late. I've found someone else and I'm happy."

"I was devastated when my husband left. But now I'm seeing someone, I am in love, and I am

loved and respected. He sees who I am, not my body, even if it sags horribly. I feel for the first time in my life, that I have found someone who sees who I am."

"I'm happy. I'm healthy. I'm single and fine with that. I actually danced with my son last night in the living room and he wore out before I did. Life is good."

It gets down to whether your spouse loved you or your weight. If your spouse loved the person inside the weight, then the love will endure. If your spouse loved the weight and the impact it had on your personality, then the marriage's demise is probably inevitable and ultimately is the healthiest outcome for you.

Both you and your spouse will have adjustments to make, and both of you may go a bit overboard in your initial reactions. Once the dust clears, you'll know whether the marriage is one in which you can be a healthy person, with a partner that can give you the support and love that you deserve.

You shouldn't accept any less.

CHAPTER SEVEN

Get in the Game – Dating After Bariatric Surgery

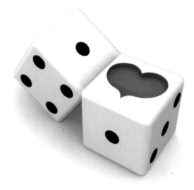

Dating. Not many words evoke such a nail-biting mix of giddiness and panic, especially for someone who's done little more than test the dating pool with their big toe. After all, people who've never had bariatric surgery don't feel like throwing up before a first date, do they?

Yes. They do.

Dating after weight loss surgery can be scary, but it's no less frightening for you than it is for anyone else. Or, to flip that around, it has the potential to be as exhilarating for you as it is for someone who's never had a weight problem.

Post-surgery patients tend to divide into five dating groups: the bench warmers, the masqueraders, the rookies, the rust buckets, and the gluttons. You'll recognize yourself in one of them.

The bench warmers never get in the game because they always hear a voice in their head saying something like, "My body looks like a wrinkled pear and I have bat wings instead of upper arms. I'll just stay home on Saturday night, swaddled in my sweats watching *Law and Order* reruns. No one's going to want to go out with me."

Baloney.

Everyone has an issue that looms in their mind as a deal killer. Their thighs are too big. Their nose is crooked. Ever since they had kids, their stomachs pooch out. They're bald. They have rosacea spots on their cheeks. Their teeth are crooked. They cut off three fingers trying to fix the lawn mower. They limp from a botched knee surgery. They've got more wrinkles than a Shar-Pei. They have varicose veins. Their legs AND arms have cellulite. Their hair is too thin and fine. They had acne as a child that scarred their faces. Their feet are too big. Their hands are too small. They went overboard with arm tattoos and now everyone can read that they joined the Marines, they love mom, and that b*!#!* Diana broke their hearts.

But, miracle of miracles, those people date. Others find them not only attractive, but flat out irresistible. Everyone knows that perfect looks exist only on retouched, airbrushed magazine covers and no one (except someone who needs to log serious time on a psychiatrist's couch) expects a perfect ten from a date.

It's really about attitude. If you like yourself, that acts as a magnet to other people. If you're proud of the way you look, others will be drawn to that confidence. Most of all, if you're genuinely interested in your date, your unwavering attention can be the most bewitching thing in the world. Imperfect people all over the world date, fall in love, and live happily (mostly) ever after.

Go ahead. Take yourself off the bench.

Let's say you're willing to get in the game, but only if you can masquerade as someone else, someone who's never had a weight problem. You view your former size and surgery as a secret so disgraceful, so shameful, that your dream date would hit the eject button if they ever found out. You've constructed a whole new self, so why does anyone have to know the awful truth about your past?

Because it's not awful. It's an integral part of who you are and something to be proud of. What you've done is an impressive accomplishment, requiring extraordinary resolve and discipline. You should be as proud of that as of telling someone you completed the Ironman Triathlon. Twice.

You don't have to spill the beans right away, but if the relationship has long term potential, you need to share the information. If you can't bring yourself to disclose your weight loss past, then that unwillingness to leave the masquerade ball is telling you something either about yourself or your chosen significant other that bears close scrutiny, because the fact that you had a weight problem significant enough to require surgery is nothing more than a small piece of personal baggage. Everyone's got at least one piece, and most have an entire matched set.

They have six children, or a bitter ex-spouse who calls constantly, or they're a recovering alcoholic, or in bankruptcy, or their son is in jail, or they've lost their job, or their nightmare of a mother lives with them, or they've been married three times, or have commitment issues, or use thirty-seven words when one would be plenty. They had an abusive childhood, or have been burned so many times they trust no one, or spend too much money, or hoard every penny, or have a serious foot fetish, or absolutely believe from the bottom of their hearts that the world will be taken over by E.T.- like aliens who will appear first in Sedona, Arizona in the year 2075.

Once the light bulb clicks on and you ferret out a daunting fact, like that your date has a shoe collection that would put Imelda Marcus to shame, you might delete that person from your contacts list, while someone else would be willing to convert their spare bedroom into a boutique style shoe closet. In other words, there's no guarantee that revealing your weight issue won't kill a potential relationship, but that's no different than anyone else's piece of baggage.

In real life, everyone has an issue or two or twenty. If your date can't deal with the fact that you used to weigh more than you do now, they're not the person for you.

Then there's the rookie, the one who's eager to play the dating game but hasn't ever been within ten miles of the arena. You've been overweight since childhood, too shy to date or maybe no one ever asked you out. You're not sure how to flirt. You're afraid of rejection. You don't know how to respond to the sudden attention you're now getting. For goodness sakes, you're not even sure how to kiss properly.

Relax.

Sure, it won't go perfectly and it won't be easy. Your dating radar will need to be calibrated. Mistakes will be made. Hearts will be broken. People will say they'll call who won't. Your best friend will steal your boyfriend. You'll steal your best friend's boyfriend. You'll fall in love on the first date. You'll fall out of love three days later. You'll obsessively phone and text the object of your affection. Someone you have no interest in will obsessively phone and text you.

In other words, all the things that would have happened had you started dating in high school will happen now. The good news is that you'll be more mature and thus able to handle the highs and lows with more aplomb than your teen self would have done. And you'll learn at supersonic speed. In a surprisingly short time, you won't even remember that you felt like a dating rookie.

Unlike the rookie, the rust bucket has been there and done that, but so long ago that the Ice Age had just barely ended. You feel like a neglected ship that's finally been hoisted out of the water into dry dock for repair only to find what looks like an impenetrable layer of rust and barnacles. You're divorced or you haven't dated in years. You've never been on eHarmony or match.com, you're not even sure what speed-dating means, and you can't text, let alone sext.

Thousands of people are in your same boat. Your experience will be no different than theirs with one important exception. You've examined your stressors in life and have taken steps to deal with them in a healthy way. You made the decision to change your life, and you know what you want. You're looking for something better and you have a pretty good idea of what that is. In that regard, you're light years ahead of most of the dating population.

Don't worry about your rustiness. It's only temporary, and your self-awareness will more than make up for it.

The final group is the gluttons, the ones who just can't get enough, typically younger people trying to catch up for their lost teens and twenties dating years in a matter of weeks. You dive headlong into the dating world without much reflection on the consequences. You'll date anyone and everyone. You're getting more attention than you've ever had, you're feeling good about yourself, you can count the number of dates you had in your pre-surgery life on one hand, so you figure, why not?

Gluttons can't push away from the Thanksgiving feast of social opportunity that has suddenly opened up for them. They fall in and out of love as frequently as they change clothes. They may not even be looking for love, but just want as many dates as possible since they've been living in the Sahara desert of dating for years.

This is normal. It won't last forever. It's like the employees who work for Mars, the M & M company. Vending machines dispense free candy all day long, and new hires feel like they've been given the keys to the Willy Wonka Chocolate Factory, binging on candy until they're sick. But after a few weeks they settle down and sample the goods in moderation.

Likewise, at some point the revolving door theory of dating won't be satisfactory anymore, and you'll settle into a more focused social scene.

What if you don't fit any of these categories? You're getting out there, using the online-dating sites and asking friends for fix-ups, but you can't get a date, or, if you do, you never get a second one.

The reason probably has nothing to do with your weight loss surgery. Maybe you're not making yourself emotionally available, or you're sending signals that you're not a happy person, or you have another piece of baggage, a big steamer trunk of an issue that's putting off potential dates.

If you're trying but aren't garnering any interest, you need to submit to an honest appraisal of what's going on, either by going to a therapist or asking for a no-holds-barred evaluation from a trusted friend or family member.

This is an exciting time. Dating is a wonderful aspect of the second chance at a healthy life you've worked so hard to get. Go out there and get in the game.

CHAPTER EIGHT

My Weight Loss Is About Me, So Why Does Everyone Act Like It's About Them?

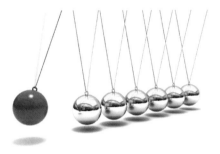

You're the one who decided to face your weight issue head on by submitting to bariatric surgery, you're the one who felt like a human petri dish while you experimented with what food your new stomach would tolerate, and you're the one who now hits the gym every night instead of the couch. You set your sights on a new life and you're doing everything you can to achieve it, a crusade as individual to you as Edmund Hillary's quest to climb Mount Everest.

So why do other people act like they have a personal stake in it?

You may have thought it was all about you, but in fact your transformation impacts every relationship you have, from your mother to your best friend to your co-workers, some with just a ripple and others with a tidal wave of repercussions.

For most, your metamorphosis will be inspiring. Bearing witness to someone else's successful struggle to change their circumstances lets everyone dare to hope they can do the same. It's why we enjoy watching movies like *Rocky* or *Miracle* or *Billy Elliot,* where ordinary people overcome Herculean obstacles to change their lot in life.

At one time or another, every adult faces the fundamental question asked by Melvin Udall, the brilliant but beleaguered obsessive compulsive character in the movie *As Good As It Gets.* Bowing to the bizarre demands of his untreated disease has boxed him into a bitter, isolated existence, finally leaving him miserable enough to confront his illness but terrified that he can't be helped. When he sees the weary faces of other patients like him sitting in his psychiatrist's waiting room, he panics and blurts out, "What if this is as good as it gets?"

Your weight loss publicly answers this universal question with a reassuring, in-your-face "not if you don't want it to be".

You didn't set out to impact everyone else – you were just trying to take care of yourself. But you did.

> *"I'm a high school teacher and had started work-*
> *ing out in a gym after school. A lot of my students*

started showing up to work out with me, and now we're training together to do a 10k."

"People at work see how I'm eating differently now and exercising. I use the myfitnesspal app to track my calories eaten and burned, and now several of them are using it too."

"My brother decided to get the [weight loss] surgery after seeing how well it worked for me."

"My ex-husband was very rude about my weight gain when we were married. We still have to deal with each other because of our son, but his attitude has now totally changed. He's willing to work with me on visitation and other things, which he's never done before. I know it's because I've lost weight."

"My daughter didn't want me to have the surgery because she said she'd be the fattest person in the house. But now she's walking with me and wanting to eat the food I eat. It's such a relief to see her wanting to be healthier."

Unfortunately, there will be a few who won't want to join the party. They were pretty comfortable with the status quo, back when you weighed more, got less attention, and didn't feel as good about yourself. You've forced them to change their view of your place in their world.

For others, you've brought their own shortcomings into unflattering focus after looking into the mirror your success has placed in front of them. They'd always thought the answer to Melvin Udall's question was "yes, this IS as good as it gets," but you've just demonstrated that momentous change is possible, exposing the soft underbelly of the excuses they've used for years to avoid facing their own personal Pandora's box of issues.

Relatives who you'd have sworn would be supportive may surprise you with their lack of enthusiasm. But think about it. You've just updated and deleted whole sections of a family operating manual that's been in place since you graduated from a crib to a bunk bed, an act that could be viewed to be as treasonous as amending the Constitution without putting it to a vote.

Let's say you've always been the focus of familial hand wringing because of your weight problem. Now who'll be the one to take your place inside the family worry box, the one everyone shakes their head over as the person who just doesn't seem to have it all together?

Or, what if you've always been the heaviest member of a family filled with weight problems. Now who gets to be the yardstick against which everyone else measures their weight with an inward sigh of relief, as in, "I may be heavy, but at least I'm not as heavy as X"? In a few families, your weight loss will cause a macabre game of musical chairs as everyone tries to avoid taking the seat you vacated.

It's not just the physical weight loss that will roil the family organizational chart. You may be noticeably more confident. You may be more assertive in your interactions with your family.

Confidence and a greater appreciation of the need to take care of yourself are hallmarks of successful bariatric patients, and sometimes it takes a while for your loved ones to adjust to the difference in the way you handle yourself. For example, if you always went along with what everyone else wanted regardless of your personal desires, your willingness to express opinions or take up for yourself may disconcert relatives who'd always taken your acquiescence for granted.

Your family's reaction to the new you can range from covert efforts to sabotage your success, to open warfare as others fight to retain their old roles and cram you back into yours, to a period of icy relations while everyone tries to absorb the changes to the now obsolete operating manual.

> *"My mom actually told me, 'I think you're a better person when you're heavier. You're not as self-absorbed.'"*

> *"My dad is overweight and just views the whole thing as a discipline problem. I don't think he'll ever approve. In his mind, I was never a disciplined person and now I've cheated by having surgery."*

> *"My parents keep telling me I'm too skinny, but I'm not even at the goal weight approved by my doctor yet. They say they're worried about me, like I've developed an eating disorder or something."*

> *"My mother won't even talk about the surgery with me. She's now gone on one of those extreme diets, and told my sister there's no way she's going to let me be smaller than her."*

"My mother and all my aunts are extremely overweight. My mom has been on some kind of a diet ever since I can remember. I thought she didn't want me to do it [the surgery] because she was afraid of the surgery itself, but I'm now six months out and I can tell she's not happy about it. I feel like I'm tiptoeing on eggshells around her."

"My sister wanted me to get the surgery, but now she says I'm just 'all about me'."

What do you do if you're on the receiving end of resentful backlash from your family? There's no silver bullet, but communication and patience are key. You may just have to give everyone time – time to adjust to your changes and time to assure themselves that the old operating manual is gone for good. There will be some growing pains, but everyone should settle down as the months pass.

If, however, the conflict continues, your family could be holding onto an unhealthy dynamic that may have contributed to your weight problem in the first place. If that's the case, don't let their behavior derail your efforts. They're really grappling with their own issues, not yours. You can't avoid your family, but you can limit time with them if it's harming your efforts to remain healthy.

A small percentage of patients used food in the past to hide from or cope with their families, either because of abuse or some other form of trauma. If you're one of these, you'll need to think carefully about how you interact with your relatives. You should seek professional help and develop a plan to deal with your family and the head hunger you're sure to feel around them. Don't kid yourself that you can handle it alone. Such deep-seated feelings will require sustained, consistent work with a competent therapist to overcome.

Friends, on the other hand, will be easier to deal with. Most will be thrilled for you. A handful may not be, however, for the same reasons that some family members may need an adjustment period – your changed role may affect theirs, and your new confidence may lead you to interact differently with them.

"So I've lost a good friend that I used to go out with. She didn't like that I am now competition. We can still talk about things like clothes, but we don't go out together anymore."

"Most of my friends are supportive. But there are some who were bigger than me and now they're not. They call me 'skinny bitch' and they're not always joking."

"Friday night I went out with some friends I've known since I was twelve. Everyone has been so amazed with my progress and so sweet. One friend, though, said, 'Just so you know, I will not let you get skinnier than me,' and she wasn't joking."

"I've been trying to get my friend to do things with me other than go out to eat. It's not working. We used to see each other every week, but I haven't seen her now in three months."

Some friendships turn out to be based almost solely on food, and once that common ground is removed there's no foundation left on which to continue. If you were the one always up for nachos and salt-rimmed margaritas at that hole-in-the-wall Tex-Mex place, you may find that your buddy is unwilling to change restaurants or try a new activity. That same friend may be one who'd never have thought of inviting you on a bike ride or hiking trip in the past and can't seem to wrap his mind around the fact that you'd like to be included now.

For those who fall away, the friendship was too shallow to survive and, although it may hurt a bit, you're much better off without them if they can't accept the new you. Besides, there's an ocean of people waiting to take their place. Your weight loss means you're up for adventure, you have the stamina to go hiking or swimming or golfing, or even shop all day. You can travel easily and you now have the energy to coach that little league team. Your world is opening up, not shrinking.

Your weight loss can lead to new opportunities at work as well.

> *"All of a sudden people knew my name who never had before. People talk to me that didn't talk to me before."*

> *"I've gotten some promotions at work, mostly I think because now I'm participating more than I did. I'm more outgoing and I volunteer to do more."*

> *"People are friendlier. They seem to respect me more."*

"I think people take me more seriously because I showed that I could commit to something and stick with it. I think I get more respect at work."

If a problem arises at work because of your weight loss, it's usually coming from your anger over being treated better than you were before, as paradoxical as that seems. Many obese people encounter discrimination every day on the job, and the extent of that intolerance may not hit home until you experience life as a "normal" person.

"A doctor at work who'd never spoken to me before started greeting me in the halls and giving me a little finger wave. It made me mad."

"An attorney who'd walked by my desk every day for years stopped and asked if I'd gotten a new haircut. I guess I'd been invisible to him before."

"One of my co-workers who sits just across the hall came up and introduced himself to me. I've been there for five years."

"All of a sudden my boss is putting me on bigger projects. Nothing's changed except my size, so it's pretty clear to me that he thinks fat people aren't as competent as thin people. I'm not okay with that."

If you're feeling angry about the change in the way others treat you, take a deep breath and give yourself some time to get used to the more welcoming environment. For the most part, your co-workers' former attitude came from ignorance or fear, and you don't have time to waste expending negative energy railing against their prejudice. Instead, use that bias that's now working in your favor to advance your career and relationships at work. After all, living well is the best revenge.

Like it or not, you've become a role model, and your change will cause the people in your orbit to examine their own lives. For the few that can't adjust, just keep in mind that the problem is about them, not you, and don't allow their negative reaction affect your continued pursuit of a healthy, full life.

CHAPTER NINE

Breaking the Three Food Commandments

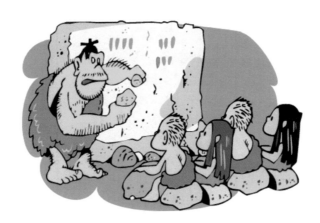

Thousands of years ago, a lightening bug drifted into a cave lit by a crude fire. A young boy followed its flickering movement, his mouth forming a small "O". He dropped the hunk of mammoth meat he'd been eating and scampered toward it.

A sinewy arm wearing a pebble bracelet grabbed the boy's wrist, yanking him back, and then reached to snatch the meat from the dirt floor. The boy stared up at his mother as she brushed the flecks of soil off the meat and then shoved it into his hand.

"What are you doing?" she said, glaring at him. "No fooling around until you finish every bite." It was at that moment, in the flickering light of the caveman's home, that the first food commandment was born.

Mothers have been saying some variation of the same thing ever since. "Clean your plate" has been hard wired into our consciousness since time began, and for good reason. When you had to hunt, grow, harvest or travel long distances to get your food, eating all that was available when it was available meant the difference between living and dying.

As the mammoths and sabre toothed tigers disappeared from the earth and man became more civilized, dessert appeared on the scene, and what kid wouldn't rather have a brownie than peas and carrots? Mothers everywhere adopted the second food commandment almost immediately: "No dessert unless you eat every bite of your meal".

After all, a person couldn't harvest corn or search for berries or hunt for wild boar if they only had empty calories in their stomachs. The commandment was also foolproof because (1) there wasn't an endless supply of food so the amount you ate would still leave room for dessert and (2) if you became full with the regular meal, you wouldn't want dessert.

As food became even more plentiful, a corollary to the dessert rule came into being, also known as the conservation commandment: "Don't eat that because it'll spoil your breakfast/lunch/supper." A scheduled meal had the nutrients you needed for hard work, and if you snacked ahead of time you wouldn't be hungry enough to consume the fuel your body needed for manual labor, which would lead to fainting dead away in the middle of the field you're trying to plow.

These three food commandments – clean your plate, no dessert unless you finish your meal, and no in-between meal snacking – have been in place for centuries. And, unlike the ten commandments brought down from Mount Sinai by Moses, the food commandments are followed religiously by most people. They've been programmed into our consciousness since our first bite of solid food.

Your mission? To break all three.

"Clean your plate" has no place in today's super-abundant food society. We won't starve to death if we don't take advantage of every meal when it's offered, and we don't need as many calories as our ancestors.

We sit at a desk or in a car, we buy food at a grocery store, and we have to schedule time to exercise because our lives don't require the level of physical exertion expended by our ancestors. "Clean your plate" is bad advice when the plate can be refilled multiple times a day and our caloric requirements are only a fraction of what great-grandpa needed to get through the day.

The easy availability of food also dooms the dessert commandment. If you plan to eat a piece of apple pie, a better rule would be to leave food on your plate so the pie won't put you over your body's caloric needs. Losing some nutritional value to indulge in dessert won't render you unable to finish your daily chores as it did two hundred years ago. On the other hand, cramming in extra calories by eating every morsel on your plate just to give yourself permission to eat more calories will send the numbers of your scale soaring in the wrong direction.

71

You're probably thinking you understand why the first two commandments have to go, but that third one about not spoiling your supper sounds pretty smart. Shouldn't it survive?

No.

Let's say you have dinner reservations at 7:30 p.m., but you're hungry at 5:00 p.m. You don't eat because "you'll spoil your supper." By the time you get to the restaurant you're ravenous. You can't wait until the bread basket arrives, and you tear into your food like you'll never see a decent meal again. Since it takes your body a minimum of ten minutes to tell you when you're full, odds are you'll be well beyond satiation by the time you get the message. The better move would have been to have a small snack. Your overall caloric intake would've remained lower and you wouldn't feel like a stuffed pig by the time after-dinner coffee arrives.

Breaking your childhood programming won't be easy. You'll eat a third of the food on your plate and put your fork down, only to hear "but children in China are starving" in your head. Or you'll be mesmerized by the piece of cheesecake sitting on the dessert cart by your table at the restaurant, and you'll feel wasteful if you don't eat every morsel of your entrée before ordering it. Or your entire family has gathered for a big Thanksgiving dinner, so you "save up" for the coming feast even though your stomach growls every five minutes.

You'll not only have to wage an internal fight with your lifelong indoctrination, you may have to battle your family and friends as well. After all, they were instructed in the same food commandments and have been following them their whole lives. They may not appreciate your disregard for the rules they view as sacrosanct. More than that, they may take it as a personal rejection.

Our society feeds one another to show love. After all, food is essential to life, so what could be more caring than feeding someone? From Jesus feeding the crowds with loaves and fishes, to the Indians sharing their food with the starving Pilgrims, to Miep Gies bringing food to Anne Frank and her family, the act of sharing food with someone is as basic and fundamental a show of affection as there is.

So when you turn down food from your family and friends, they may interpret your action as a slap at them. For most of your life, they've cooked special dinners for your birthday, taken you out to your favorite restaurant to celebrate your promotion, and brought cookies over when you're feeling down. These are all generous, loving gestures, and if you now eat sparingly or turn down the food altogether, they may interpret that as a sign that you don't love them, you don't appreciate their care, or you're being downright rude.

You'll need to explain to them why you're not eating as much, even on special occasions. You'll need to reassure them that you care for them and appreciate their care for you, either directly or by your actions.

You may get some push back, as in snide comments like, "I'd take you out, but you won't eat anyway so what's the point."

Don't take the bait. Be patient and give them a little time to accept your new behavior and figure out a different way to demonstrate their love for you other than the one they've been using for years. Whatever you do, don't let guilt push you back into following the outdated food commandments.

Finally, cast a skeptical eye over the wave of modern food rules that hit the internet on a weekly basis. You know the ones – things like "no eating after 5:00 p.m." or "don't eat anything white" or "drink 64 ounces of beet juice every day". The axioms may or may not be true, but even if they are, they may not work well for you.

For example, we've been told for years that breakfast is the most important meal of the day. A recent study, however, has shown that people who skipped breakfast and worked out in the morning burned more fat and maintained their weight better than people who ate breakfast and worked out later in the day. So what do you do if you're a morning exerciser? If you can't get through a workout without breakfast, then eat your oatmeal. If you can exercise without eating breakfast first, then skip it.

Bottom line? You need to create your own rules based on what works best for you. Here are some basic commandments that you can build from:

1. Keep track of your calories, in writing, both eaten and burned.
2. Be aware what you're eating – don't graze mindlessly.
3. Don't let others dictate your meal plan.

Fighting what society has programmed into you since birth can be difficult and will require you, at times, to fly in the face of what your friends and family believe to be the gospel truth. But just remind yourself that the three food commandments were developed for a far different time and are as outdated as stone axes, hoop skirts, and rotary phones.

Be a rebel. Break the three food commandments and create new ones of your own.

CHAPTER TEN

Breaking Up with Your Ex For Good: The Maintenance Grind

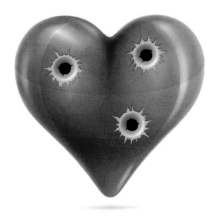

The thing about torrid love affairs is they never end with a clean break. Sure, you have every reason to think it's over. You changed your phone number, attended a weekly support group, burned every picture of the two of you together and started dating a healthier, saner person - one your friends actually like.

But passionate romances don't die until the second or third bullet. There's always at least one steamy reconciliation before the thing is finally stone cold dead.

You'll run into your ex at the store and go a little weak at the knees, or you'll send a gushing e-mail on a lonely Friday night, or you'll decide that avoidance is childish and the grownup thing to do is at least be friends. Before you know it, you're right back where you were, and after the initial exhilaration dies you realize your mistake. Nothing's really changed and you've wasted time and emotion yet again on someone who isn't and never will be good for you.

An unhealthy relationship with food is eerily similar, and breaking it off can be as difficult as Dan's struggle to get away from Alex in the movie *Fatal Attraction*.

You may be stunned to learn that you're so in love with the simple act of eating. One of the most common things bariatric surgeons hear on follow-up visits is, "I never realized what a relationship I had with food". You thought your weight problem was from ignorance over what to eat, or faulty childhood messaging, or not making time to care for yourself, or your grandmother's genes.

That may be where it started, but that's not what kept it going.

After surgery, you figure out the truth. You've been embedded in a romance as sticky and hard to leave as Richard Burton and Elizabeth Taylor's on-again-off-again love affair.

But, you say, that's all in the past. I don't even get hungry any more. I don't think about food like I used to. I'm a healthy lifestyle convert and I'm never going back. I broke up with that loser once and for all.

No, you didn't.

Just like lovers in a doomed romance, you'll be tempted to drift back into your old relationship with food. And it'll sneak up on you when you're most vulnerable, right when you think you've got the whole thing whipped.

Here's what happens. Your surgery gave you a massive head start. It forced you to change your eating habits, it did away with your hunger pangs and allowed you to drop weight at breathtaking speed. You got positive reinforcement from the immediate success of your new behavior and from the fact that you just flat out felt better. You've been working through the changed relationships with friends and family, bolstered by plunging scale numbers. You're elated every time you try on a smaller pants size and can button the waistband with room to spare. People who'd never spoken to you before, from your dry cleaner to your grocery clerk to the neighbor down the street, have raved over how great you look and have marveled at your discipline. Every week contains a little drama in the form of unaccustomed praise, changed relationships, different activities, and new clothes.

But the drama will end. The excitement from all the changes in your family and work relationships will wane. People will get used to your slimmer self and won't feel the need to compliment you anymore. Life will settle down, just like someone who's had a thrilling engagement with lots of gifts, a fabulous wedding, an extended honeymoon, and the first couple of scary post-marriage fights and rapturous make-up sessions, but now has to get used to day-to-day married life with the spouse who leaves a trail of potato chips in his wake and the mother-in-law who calls three times a day. In other words, life will become normal, and, at times, even mundane.

Even more sobering, your body will adapt over time. You'll be able to undo the straitjacket put on your system by the surgery.

For those who had a gastric bypass or vertical sleeve operation, two things come into play that will test your resolve. First, you'll get hungry again. Even though the surgery bypassed ghrelin, the hunger hormone, other hormones will ramp up to fill the void, and most patients will start feeling hungry again, anywhere from six to twenty-four months after the surgery.

Second, your new stomach will adjust and toughen up, just like babies' feet callous as they learn to walk. Your stomach will expand a bit, and its cells will change to create more and thicker mucus which cushions the food you ingest, making it easier to eat bigger quantities and varieties of food.

If you had the gastric bypass surgery, a third issue will come into play. The dumping syndrome that's kept you from eating sugar will disappear in most patients. So the piece of cake that would have made you violently ill six months ago won't cause a problem now.

For lap band patients, two issues can lure you back into your old lifestyle. First, you've figured out how to cheat, and you're familiar enough with the band that you're no longer worried about hurting yourself if you thwart its restriction. You can drink high calorie milk shakes or put your favorite food in a blender and eat as much as you want.

Second, you rely on the lap band to limit your food intake like a surgical shock collar rather than taking control of your own behavior, creating a negative reinforcement method of diet control that starts to grate on you. You have your surgeon decrease the saline in your lap band for special occasions, like Thanksgiving, and then put in enough saline "to make me throw up" when you want to lose more weight instead of taking the steering wheel and driving your own eating and exercise plan. Over time, you'll begin to resent the choke hold the band has over your body and you'll grow tired of the twice-monthly maintenance visits to your doctor.

That's why the first six months after your operation should be treated like a sprint, wringing every benefit you can from the surgery while you've got all its mechanical and behavioral benefits going for you – the compliments, the falling scale numbers, the lack of appetite, and the physical inability to eat too much. This time won't last forever, and those six months will be the best shot most people ever get at losing their excess weight.

You'll learn to listen to your body to tell you when you need food. You'll figure out what it feels like when your glucose is low, which means you need energy and should put some fuel in your tank. You'll be able to tell the difference between real hunger versus head hunger, between needing energy and just mindlessly following an eating habit, between desiring food versus needing food.

Have you ever watched *The Biggest Loser* television show? The idea behind it is great, but the recidivism rate is depressingly high. Once the cameras, personal trainers, television audience and attention go away, many contestants can't keep the weight off. Why? Because they were losing weight on a reality show that removed them from the reality of their daily lives. They never had the opportunity to develop new habits in their own environment.

You'll be given a much better chance at meeting your goals because you'll be learning to listen to your body and employing new habits in the everyday normalcy of your real life.

The maintenance mindset is different than what you're used to. It requires consistency and vigilance even when there's no positive reinforcement other than the satisfaction you get of seeing the scale number remain the same when you weigh yourself. It becomes all about the little things.

You know that ten pounds you can gain in a year by just eating a hundred extra calories a day above your needs? That's the kind of detail you need to pay attention to. The deciding factor in whether you maintain your weight loss or gain it all back boils down to simple things like burning off 200 calories every day with exercise, settling into the daily grind of eating the right foods, saying no to your trigger foods, and paying attention to every calorie you're putting in your mouth and how many calories you're burning.

There is no finish line. There is no moment when you can say, okay, I've won that battle and I can forget about it. It will require your attention every day of every week of every year. Like a recovering alcoholic has to pay attention to what he drinks for the rest of his life, you've got to be vigilant about diet and exercise for the rest of yours.

But, you say, that sounds depressing. Surely life wasn't meant to be quite so restrictive. That's just too hard.

Actually, it's not. It's just conducting yourself in a fashion that's consistent with your goals, something you've been doing your entire life with your job, your marriage, your family, and your friends.

Think about it.

Once you decided you wanted to be in a certain profession, you put in the hours of education and training to get there, went after the job you wanted, and finally got it on your second or third or eighth try. But you can't sleep in every morning or stay home watching daytime television and expect to hang onto that dream job. You've got to show up every day and perform to keep it.

Most of us accept the restriction of going to work every day, dream job or not, without thinking twice. It's a necessary part of life, if for no other reason than to pay the bills.

Or let's say you met the love of your life and finally got married after a three year courtship. Do you then put a check by "get married" on your to-do list and go back to living the way you did when you were single? Not if you want to stay married.

Sure, you could view the whole marriage thing as restrictive - and it is. You can't sleep with anyone else, you have to call home when you're going to be late, you can't take off on a vacation with your buddies without some serious negotiations, and you've got to compromise on things like budgets and chores and child-rearing. In other words, you behave in a way that allows you to keep the love of your life because the marriage is more important than the stuff you're missing out on.

The things you're proudest of in life are the things that have required the greatest work and sacrifice - your education, your children, your marriage, your career. Maintaining a healthy weight is no different and it's something you should pat yourself on the back every day for doing.

You've tasted what life is like without the suffocating excess weight. Your new habits are far less restrictive than the physical, social and emotional limitations your old weight burdened you with.

It's time to kick your dysfunctional romance with food out of your life forever.

CHAPTER ELEVEN

I'm Doing Everything Right, So Why Doesn't My Weight Show It?

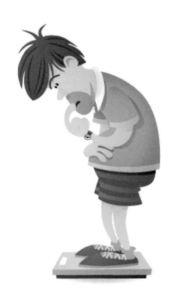

You're monitoring your calorie intake, it feels like you eat less than anyone you know, and you exercise three to four times a week. So why are you gaining weight?

"I weigh about thirty pounds more than I did at my lowest weight two years ago. I'm so frustrated. I'm doing the things I'm supposed to do but nothing seems to make a difference."

"I watch other people eating stuff I wouldn't even touch now, but I'm the one buying bigger clothes while they're doing just fine."

Many patients regain twenty to thirty pounds of the weight they lost even though they're following a reasonably healthy lifestyle. Figuring out why doesn't take the reincarnation of Sherlock Holmes, just a clear-eyed application of Occam's Razor.

Medieval philosopher William of Ockham lived in a time when almost everyone had a whispered tale to share of supernatural intervention by God or Satan or some forgotten deity striving for recognition in a world full of miracles. Ockham suspected that the spectral world might be getting a nudge from some enterprising earthlings, so he developed Occam's Razor to separate the truly divine from the shrewd flimflam.

The deceptively straightforward theory states that the simplest explanation for an event is usually the right one. Occam's Razor solved mysteries like whether the red lines streaking down the face of the Virgin Mary statue were remnants of bloody tears or berry stains daubed on by a misguided monk trying to raise enough money to fix the abbey's leaky roof.

In modern times, Occam's Razor solves a variety of logic questions. If, for example, the candy bar you left on your desk is missing and your six-year-old has chocolate smeared on his face, you'll most likely believe he ate it, no matter how many times he insists that a UFO small enough to fit through a window flew into the room and sucked it up with a magnetic laser beam.

Occam's Razor says you can't squeeze into the pants you wore six months ago because you ate more calories than you burned. So what's the simplest explanation for the calorie disparity?

It's usually one or more of three possible culprits.

First, you may have lost the dedicated zeal you had in your first few months or years following surgery. You focused hard on your own health after your surgery and now you've shifted your attention to other things and have become a bit less rigid about your diet and exercise.

Maybe you've been grazing during the day more than you realize, or you've added ice cream back into your repertoire now that your dumping syndrome is gone, or you're not as careful when you go out to eat as you once were. Maybe you only work out three times a week when a year ago your gym's Stairmaster practically had your name engraved on it.

It won't be hard to figure out. Take a clear-eyed look at your habits and compare them to what you were doing before you gained the twenty or thirty pounds. If you haven't already, begin keeping a food and exercise journal and review it carefully. You'll find your weight gain culprit.

Second, you may be a victim of slowing metabolism. The average patient walks into their bariatric surgeon's office around their fortieth birthday, which means they begin their weight loss war on a battlefield of increasingly unfavorable conditions.

The rate of metabolism slows in your early forties, and then falls off a cliff between ages forty-five to fifty. If you're in that milestone decade, your body's slowing metabolic rate explains why you're eating and expending the same amount of calories you were a year ago but your weight keeps creeping up. You've got to eat less, exercise more, or do both.

Before you fall into a blue funk over the unfairness of it all, keep in mind that you've now landed in the world of mainstream weight problems. Slowing metabolism happens to everyone, even people who never had to worry about their weight before. You'll have lots of company in finding the right strategies to keep your weight down as you age.

Third, you may have succumbed to the success phenomenon. Many bariatric patients find themselves on the fast track at work, their career soaring to unexpected heights because of their weight loss and increased self-confidence. The impact of success on weight (unless you're a professional athlete) can be predicted almost to a mathematical certainty:

Promotion

+

Increased Pay

+

More Responsibility

↓

Less Energy Expended

↓

WEIGHT GAIN

Why? You get a closer parking space so you don't burn the hundred calories you once did by parking in the boonies and walking up the stairs in the parking garage. Someone now gets your files for you and people come to your office instead of you walking to theirs. You're spending longer hours sitting behind a desk or studying your computer screen. You can afford expensive wine at dinner now instead of iced tea. Someone else mows your lawn, cleans your house, walks your dog and washes your windows.

Remember the ten pounds a year just a hundred extra calories a day adds to your frame? Your very success may have resulted in small changes in your normal routine that, over time, led to the twenty or thirty pounds you've been unable to shed.

If none of these three applications of Occam's Razor explains your weight gain, then it's time to call in the professionals. Go see your bariatric surgeon and give a candid explanation of what's going on, not only with your weight, but with your life. Between the two of you, you'll find the answer for the cause of your weight gain, and can develop a plan to get you back to where you want to be.

Your weight gain isn't inexplicable and doesn't have to be permanent. You've already shown you can lose weight and keep it off. Once you figure out the reasons you've lost some ground, you can make the appropriate changes and get back to where you want to be.

CHAPTER TWELVE

When to Declare Victory: Managing Expectations

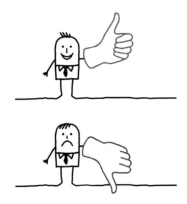

Most people contemplating bariatric surgery have one goal in mind: getting healthy. Sure, a few delusional souls want the moon and the stars in the form of losing a hundred pounds in three months so they can wow their old high school friends at the twenty year reunion, but the average patient simply wants a normal life.

They temper their expectations, their voices sliding up in a question when the surgeon asks about their weight loss goals, fearful of being laughed at. They're shocked when the doctor tells them what they can achieve using the surgery as a tool.

"When my surgeon told me my goal weight was 175 pounds, I thought he was nuts. The last time I weighed 175 pounds was in eighth grade, almost thirty years ago. If I could get down to 250 pounds I'd think that was a miracle."

"My doctor told me I won't live five more years if I don't get the weight off. I don't really think the goal my surgeon recommended is possible, but if that'll get rid of my diabetes I'll give it my best shot."

But then things change.

Pounds drop off, you start feeling better and you now know that the weight you thought was a pipe dream just months before is actually doable. So you move the goal line, raising or lowering your expectations, and nine times out of ten the direction of the shift is gender based. Yes, the whole *Men are From Mars, Women are From Venus* thing kicks in even in the area of bariatric surgery.

If you're a woman, what would have been satisfactory a year ago isn't good enough. Before the surgery, you were only worried about getting healthy to take care of your family. You'd have been thrilled to fit into a size 10, something that seemed as unlikely to you as being the cover girl for the *Sports Illustrated* swimsuit edition.

Now you'll only be satisfied if you can wear a size 4 or 2. You're unhappy with your appearance in a way you never were before, and you're convinced you look worse than you did before the surgery because at least your skin didn't fold over on itself like it does now. You're saving your money for plastic surgery, not just for your excess skin, but for a boob job, an eye lift or maybe even a full facelift. Your emotional focus becomes increasingly on how you look, not on how you physically feel.

Remember Lucy yanking the football away just as Charlie Brown is about to kick it, landing him flat on his back? You're playing the part of both Lucy *and* Charlie Brown. Just like Lucy is never going to let Charlie Brown kick the ball, you're never going to allow yourself to put a check mark in the weight loss win column. You've forgotten your original goal – to get healthier – and are consumed with your looks.

If you're a man, the goal your surgeon set at the beginning now seems like overkill, not because you can't reach it but because you've met your original goal of getting healthier. Even though you only lost fifty pounds when your surgeon recommended you lose a hundred, your diabetes or your high blood pressure or your sleep apnea – the health crisis that drove you to get bariatric surgery – is gone. You're happy where you are. You got the ball down to the forty yard line and went ahead and called it a touchdown.

Why the difference between the sexes? Society's centuries-old pressure on women to fit a specific, and, in today's waif-worshiping world, almost impossible physical image contrasted against its more tolerant view of acceptable male physiques. Most men don't feel unattractive over a volley-ball-sized paunch while a woman might feel like a beached whale over a small muffin top.

Even though the men may be underperforming, they're correct. They've won. They could win by a wider margin if they lost more weight, but a win is a win, whether by one point or twenty.

Bariatric surgery's purpose is to lower high blood pressure, cure diabetes, stop liver disease, slow down the progress of degenerative joint disease, alleviate the need for a knee or other joint replacement, ease the stress on your back, and lower your weight to a size your heart can handle, staving off future cardiac problems. Any improvement in your looks from the weight loss is a nice bonus, but shouldn't obscure the progress you've made in the area that really counts – your health.

So how do you keep focused on realistic expectations? Think back to what you said the first time you walked into your surgeon's office.

> *"I've got diabetes. My aunt died of it, after having toes and a foot amputated. I'm scared to death that's going to happen to me."*

> *"I just want to be healthy. I want to live to see my grandchildren grow up."*

> *"I want to be able to ski, ride a bicycle, go fishing – do things I used to do but can't anymore."*

> *"My doctor told me my weight would kill me if I didn't do something about it. That woke me up."*

"I'm sick and tired of sleeping with a CPAP machine and taking high blood pressure medication."

"It's gotten to the point that I can't even play with my kids anymore because I get too out of breath. I want to do things with them like normal dads do with their sons."

"My daughter isn't at a healthy weight for her age. When her pediatrician told me, he looked almost embarrassed and I knew what he was thinking. How could I do anything about my daughter's weight when my own is so out of control? I've got to set a better example."

Write down those initial goals and keep them handy. They'll remind you of how far you've come and can be a good measuring stick by which to evaluate whether your current expectations are reasonable. If you got rid of the health problems that plagued you before the surgery that's a win, no matter what pants size you wear.

A simple way to check the appropriateness of your expectations is to examine them in terms of "want" versus "need". For example, you need to get rid of your diabetes or high blood pressure or liver disease. You may want to wear a size 4 dress to your sister's wedding. Don't let your "wants" rob you of the epic triumph of having met your "needs".

Some people, both male and female, have a different issue than declaring victory too early or too late. They can't make a call one way or the other because their perceptions have been skewed from years of seeing themselves as overweight.

These people fall into two categories: the ones who need a new prescription for their mental eyeglasses, and the ones who got the new prescription but don't like what they see.

If you're in the first category, your brain doesn't believe what your eyes reflect in the mirror. You go to the plus size section of the department store even though none of those clothes fit you anymore. Your BMI chart is in the normal range, the scale says you're at or below your goal weight, but you're sure the scale is wrong or the surgeon miscalculated because you don't look any different than you always have. While your friends see someone who looks dramatically different, you see yourself as looking the same. This is a normal reaction, particularly for people who've been overweight most of their lives.

Your brain will adjust to your new look, just like your eyes adjust over time to your first set of progressive bifocals. In the meantime, you can help it along by doing things like checking your clothes size compared to the size you used to wear, or taking pictures of yourself and comparing them to old photos. The longer you've been overweight, the longer this stage can last, but your mind will learn to see you as you really are over time.

On the opposite end of the spectrum are the people who can see just fine, and that's the problem. They can't get comfortable with their changed physical image. They expected to be happier once they lost weight, but instead they're depressed and anxiety-ridden, disconcerted by the stranger looking back at them in the mirror. They feel they don't know who they are anymore, which may lead them to start gaining weight just to get back to the person they recognize.

If you're one of these people, talk to your surgeon and tell him/her what's going on. Your doctor can refer you to a therapist who will give you the help you need in matching your new body to your old identity.

You've done something momentous and changed your life forever. Pat yourself on the back and take the win. You've earned it.

CHAPTER THIRTEEN

Revision Surgery – You Don't Want to Go There

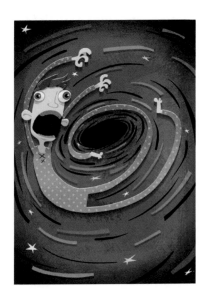

The best revision surgery is the one that never happens. Getting it right the first time is not only your best chance at weight loss, it may be your only chance.

Imagine being born blind, miraculously gaining your sight through cutting edge surgery, discovering a glorious world of vibrant colors, and then having your newfound vision ripped away. That's how some bariatric surgery patients describe the exhilaration of losing weight and the agony of gaining it all back. They've experienced life as a normal person and now know with pinpoint clarity what a handicap their weight is. Some wish they'd remained "blind", feeling it would have been less painful to have never lost the weight at all.

> *"Before the surgery, I suspected people might be treating me differently because of my weight. Now that I've lost and gained it all back, I know they do."*

> *"I used to think people treated me the way they did because I was fifty, but it was really because I was fat."*

Patients who end up back where they started before the surgery wear a hair shirt of mortification, disillusion and pure panic. Not only do they feel like failures, but they've seen through an unfiltered lens the view normal-sized people have of obese people and can never look at the world quite the same again. So it's no surprise that they want a do-over, pronto.

But bariatric surgery is rarely better the second time around. Why? Because the first bariatric surgery is like being presented with a shiny new tool box with state of the art devices all designed to work together to help you lose weight, while revision surgery is more like strapping on a battered tool belt jangling with worn out gadgets, none of which are exactly the tools you need.

Whether revision surgery will be successful for you depends primarily on why the initial surgery failed.

The first thing your doctor will investigate is whether the mechanical aspects of the initial surgery worked as they should have. In other words, he'll check to see if the procedure was performed correctly, and, even if it was, whether a subsequent mechanical failure thwarted the weight loss benefits the surgery was supposed to provide. Mechanical problems are usually fixable, and once corrected the patient can lose down to a healthy weight and maintain it.

If you're one of these people, revision surgery is a good option for you.

Other patients regain the weight they lost because they were derailed by some major life change. They started out doing exactly what they were supposed to do, working hard at the behavioral changes necessary for success, but then something big happened - good or bad - that caught them flat-footed. Their child got leukemia, or they started traveling more when they got the promotion at work, or they had to care for an elderly parent, or they married a wealthy person and had access to things they never had before. Their dedication to a healthier game plan went out the window in the wake of some unanticipated life development.

These people have reasonable odds of success at revision surgery because they get it. They understand what's required for success and they've actually put it into practice for some period of time. Even though the second surgery won't provide them with as many effective tools as they originally had, it can still provide enough help to get them to a healthy weight for good.

The final and most common reason for regaining weight after bariatric surgery is that the patient never bought into the behavioral changes needed for the operation to work. These people viewed the surgery as a passive process, as something that would "fix" them, like having an appendix removed.

They lost weight for six months and then gained it all back because they counted on the procedure to change their behavior instead of working at it themselves. Once the temporary effects of the surgery wore off – the ghrelin suppression, the inability to eat too much, the dumping syndrome – they went back to their old lifestyle and regained the weight. Before long, they're back in their surgeon's waiting room, begging for another surgery to return them to the halcyon days of early weight loss. But even the Albert Einstein of bariatric surgeons can't do that.

If your initial surgery provided ghrelin suppression which alleviated your hunger, other hormones have up-regulated to compensate, and those can't be suppressed. If you had a procedure which resulted in dumping syndrome, your body has adapted and you can eat sweets with no adverse consequences. And mentally? You know without a doubt that you can undo the surgery since you've done it before. While some bariatric patients are terrified they'll cause themselves physical harm if they eat too much or indulge in the wrong food, you know eating your way out of your surgery won't kill you – at least not immediately.

Your toolbox has been decimated.

Sure, there are some things that can be done - the opening to your stomach or sleeve can be tightened and it's possible that the pouch can be reduced somewhat - but the mechanical aspects won't be as good as the first time around.

And, let's face it. If you didn't make the behavioral changes required with the first surgery, odds are you won't with the revised version either.

Unfortunately, there are a few surgeons who will take advantage of the desperation of patients who've regained their weight. They'll perform a useless operation on your stomach when it's really your head that needs to be fixed, or they'll recommend an extreme surgery that may leave you malnourished and plagued by other physical problems for the rest of your life.

If you're contemplating revision surgery for any reason other than a mechanical problem, invest time in seeing a therapist who specializes in weight loss issues to make sure you're prepared for it. Get a second or third opinion from other bariatric surgeons, and be cautious about agreeing to any extreme form of bariatric surgery. Unless your life is in immediate danger, that type of surgery is rarely appropriate.

You don't ever want to be in the position of contemplating revision surgery. Be proactive if you find yourself getting off track after bariatric surgery. Don't wait until you've gained all your weight back to tackle the issue. Instead, tell your doctor what's going on in your life so that he/she can steer you in the right direction before things get out of hand.

You should approach bariatric surgery as though it is your last chance to get healthy, because it probably is.

CHAPTER FOURTEEN

How to Choose Your Bariatric Surgeon

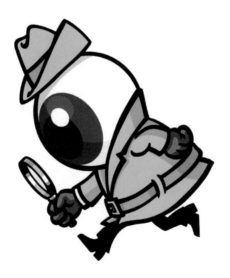

Bariatric surgeons seem to be sprouting on nearly every street corner so there's plenty to choose from, yet some people spend more time buying a car than they do in selecting the doctor who'll cut them open and perform life-altering surgery.

Don't be one of those people.

Do your research and see at least two or three surgeons before you make your decision, because the person you choose will be in your life for years and can make or break your weight loss efforts.

Picking the right one is easy if you follow these simple rules.

First, your surgeon should have done at least 1000 bariatric surgeries. If they haven't, scratch them off your list.

Second, check with the state medical board where you live to ensure that the physician is licensed. The Federation of State Medical Boards has a listing of addresses and telephone numbers for all state medical boards here: http://www.fsmb.org/directory_smb.html. For a nominal fee, the Federation will also provide you with information on whether a specific doctor's license has ever been revoked or suspended and whether he/she has ever been the subject of disciplinary action here: http://s1.fsmb.org/docinfo/. If there's no record of the doctor or you learn that they've had problems in their past, move onto the next candidate.

Third, read online reviews. Although anyone can write a review and some cranky impossible-to-please person may bash a surgeon, you shouldn't ignore numerous bad reviews, especially those that seem to have a common thread of complaint.

Fourth, interview the entire practice. Is the receptionist friendly, does the nutritionist treat you with care, is the physician's assistant competent? You'll most likely be dealing with your doctor's staff as much as the doctor, so you need to feel comfortable with them. If you're a new patient and you feel like you're in a cattle call, how do you think you'll be treated when you call at two in the morning trying to get through to your physician? If the whole practice doesn't treat you with compassion, competence and respect, then move on.

Fifth, don't rely exclusively on your general practitioner's recommendation. Most are competent to say other patients have had a good experience with a certain doctor, but they aren't competent to say how they act at the hospital. Your g.p. may not know if a particular surgeon throws things in the operating room, treats their staff with disrespect that then bleeds down to the patient, or views their patients as just one more surgery in a volume practice instead of a person with a name and unique problems. The g.p.'s recommendation can be a good starting point, but shouldn't be the end of your inquiry.

Sixth, check out whether the practice meets the expectations it created. When you went for your appointment, did you see who you thought you were going to see or were you fobbed off onto someone else? Were your questions answered or were you rushed through the process? If anything feels fishy to you, walk away.

Seventh, if, and only if, more than one doctor meets the basic criteria outlined above, go with the one that makes you feel the most comfortable. Just like a woman who hates men should never go to a male gynecologist, you shouldn't choose someone who makes you feel uneasy. You won't trust what they say, which will add an extra level of difficulty to an already arduous task.

If you want someone who reminds you of your grandfatherly childhood doctor, you'll never have confidence in a younger doctor no matter how competent or highly recommended they are. If you can't trust a doctor unless he/she wears a white coat and uses big words, you won't be as likely to listen to one who uses simple words combined with a down-to-earth manner. If you believe that only Ivy League medical schools turn out competent physicians, you won't be happy with a doctor who graduated from a state medical school.

It doesn't matter whether the personal characteristics you prefer are right or wrong, logical or illogical, politically correct or not. You're about to engage in a long-term, committed relationship, and if you don't take your own personal likes and dislikes into account, the relationship will be handicapped from the start, which is no way to start a weight loss journey.

Once you've applied these seven rules, you'll find the doctor who can give you the best shot at meeting your goals. Approach your selection with as much care as you'd apply to selecting the right pediatrician for your only child. After all, you're the one with the life on the line.

CHAPTER FIFTEEN

Things Your Mama Should Have Told You

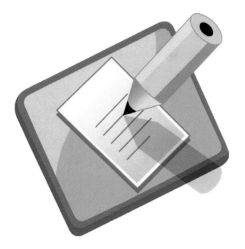

On weight loss surgery:
- There's no shame in asking for medical help for a physical problem.
- It isn't the easy way out. Anyone who tells you it is should be quietly written off as ignorant.

- You're going to have to work hard for the surgery to be successful.
- It's safer to have weight loss surgery than to remain morbidly obese.
- If you decide not to have weight loss surgery, how you feel today is probably as good as it gets.

On gaining weight:
- Most people have a perfectly normal thyroid.
- There is no such thing as a "glandular" problem.
- You can't gain weight just by looking at a chocolate cupcake. There's always a logical reason, which usually boils down to eating too much and exercising too little.

On fretting over your post-surgery body:
- No one looks good naked after a certain age.
- That age is usually at least one year younger than you are unless you're a movie star, genetically blessed, have a full time chef and trainer, a plastic surgeon on speed dial, and only have photos taken with a soft lens.
- Spanx works.
- You won't look like Angelina Jolie no matter how much weight you lose. Even Angelina Jolie doesn't look like Angelina Jolie.
- You did this for your health, not to look better.

On food:
- If your grandmother wouldn't recognize that thing you're about to put in your mouth as food, you shouldn't either.

- Shelf life for food is like a prison term. The longer it is, the worse it is for you.
- Junk food is just that – junk. Don't eat it.
- Your taste buds become sensitized after the first bite, so the first bite is the best bite. Everything after that is mostly your imagination.
- Watching your diet isn't restrictive. It's liberating.
- You don't need a Ph.D. in nutrition to lose weight. It's just calories in and calories out.

On exercise:
- Exercise doesn't require a gym membership.
- Nowhere does it say you have to love exercise to do it.
- Little things count as exercise such as walking your dog, climbing the stairs instead of taking the elevator, walking from the parking lot into your office building, speed walking through the mall comparing prices, pacing while you talk on the phone, and weeding the garden.
- If you don't like exercise, treat it like cleaning house before company comes over - just a necessary chore that has to be done - and move on.

And finally…
- Losing weight isn't easy, but then nothing worth doing ever is. This is your one and only life. Shape it into what you want it to be.
- You can do this